CALENDULA

MARIAN KIM

ISBN: 1508561850

ISBN-13: 978-1508561859

CONTENTS

1

PROPERTIES

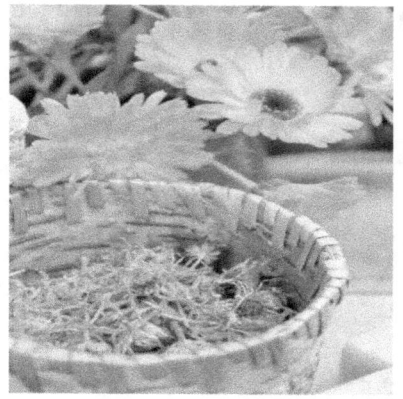

Scientific name: Calendula officinalis

Other names: Pot marigold or marigold

Properties

The properties of calendula include:

Anti-inflammatory properties

Anti-oxidant properties which protect the skin cells from free radical damage

Antiseptic (antibacterial, antiviral, antifungal,) properties

Skin soothing properties

Moisturizing properties

Tissue regenerating properties

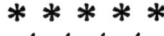

2

USES

Acne

Calendula has anti-inflammatory properties which are useful for managing the inflammation associated with acne. It also has antiseptic (antibacterial) properties which are also useful for treating acne. Calendula also has tissue regenerating properties, skin soothing and moisturizing properties and which are useful for the healing process.

Eczema

Calendula has anti-inflammatory properties which are useful for managing the inflammation associated with eczema. It also has skin soothing properties and moisturizing properties which help relieve the dryness associated with eczema. Calendula also has tissue regenerating properties and which are useful for healing of the skin.

Psoriasis treatment

Anti-inflammatory properties and acts as a soothing agent which reduces inflammation when applied to the skin. It is thus used to manage inflamed skin conditions like psoriasis. It is also used to manage psoriasis prone scalps

Dry skin moisturization

The moisturizing properties of calendula are useful for managing dry skin and chapped nipples in breastfeeding women.

Sensitive skin soother

The skin soothing properties of calendula are useful for calming sensitive skin.

Mature skin and prematurely aging skin

The antioxidant properties and tissue regenerating properties of calendula are useful for preventing premature aging and managing mature skin.

Minor cuts and wounds healer

The antibacterial and antiviral properties of calendula are useful for treating mild skin infections, wounds, minor cuts, bruises and insect bites.

Fungal infections treatment

The antifungal properties of calendula are useful for treating athlete's foot, ringworms and jock itch.

Burns

The tissue regenerating properties of calendula are useful for treating first degree burns, sunburns and scalds.

Diaper rash

Calendula oil is used for managing diaper rash which is also known as diaper dermatitis.

Chemotherapy dermatitis prevention

Calendula has been shown to prevent dermatitis or skin inflammation in breast cancer patients receiving radiation treatment.

Varicose veins treatment

Calendula is used for the treatment of varicose veins and spider veins.

Hemorrhoid treatment

Calendula is used for the treatment of hemorrhoids.

Wounds

Calendula makes a healing wash with antiseptic (antibacterial, antiviral, antifungal) properties that disinfects wounds. Its immunnostimulant properties helps poorly healing leg ulcers and wounds heal. Calendula also stimulates collagen production and minimizes scarring. It also reduces the pain and inflammation when applied to skin lesions.

Dry Scalps

Calendula is used to moisturize dry scalps.

Itchy scalps relief

Calendula infusion can be used to manage itchy scalps

Damaged hair management

Calendula conditions the hair and is useful for managing heat and sun damaged hair.

Muscle sprains relief

Calendula is used to manage sprains and bruises. It is also used to prevent muscle spasms.

Start menstruation

Calendula is used to start menstruation.

Menstrual cramps relief

Calendula is used to relieve menstrual cramps.

Fever reducer

Calendula is used to reduce fevers.

Sore throat relief

Calendula infusion is used as a gargle to relieve sore throats.

Duodenal ulcer treatment

Calendula is used to treat duodenal ulcers.

* * * * *

3

SAFETY PRECAUTIONS

1. Do not use calendula if you are allergic to it or allergic to daisy or aster family plants like ragweed and chrysanthemums.

2. Do not use calendula if you are pregnant or breastfeeding or trying to conceive.

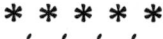

4

DRUG INTERACTIONS

Avoid calendula preparations if you are taking:

1. Sedatives

2. High blood pressure medications

3. Diabetes medications

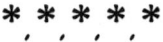

5

TIP

If you grow your own calendula, pull the petals from the flower head because you only need the petals. After plucking out the petals keep the flower heads which have now become seed heads to plant.

* * * * *

6

HERBAL RECIPES

Calendula Infusion

Equipment

Glass jar with tight fitting lid

***

Ingredients

1 tablespoon dried calendula or 3 tablespoons fresh calendula

1 cup boiling water

***

Instructions

1. Place the calendula in the glass jar and add the boiling water to fill the jar.

2. Close the lid and let the mixture steep for 4 hours to 14 hours (overnight).

3. Strain the herb and the infusion is ready for consumption.

***

Tips

1. Store the infusion in the refrigerator to lengthen its life.

2. This calendula infusion is perfect a perfect face wash for acne treatment.

3. This calendula infusion can also be used to cleanse eczema lesions.

*****

Calendula Tincture

Equipment

Glass jar with tight fitting lid

Dark tincture bottles

Cheesecloth

Labels

***

Ingredients

7 oz (200 gm) of dried herbs or 14 oz (400 gm) of fresh herbs

30 oz (1 liter) of 80-100 proof vodka

***

Instructions

1. Fill 1/3 of the glass jar with the chopped herbs.

2. Add the vodka to completely fill the jar to the top.

3. Seal the jar and label it with the date of preparation and name of herb used.

4. Store the glass jar in a dark place for 6 weeks ensuring that you shake them weekly.

5. After 6 weeks strain out the herbs with a cheesecloth and pour the tincture into dark tincture bottles.

6. Label the tincture bottles with the date and name of herb used.

7. Store your herbal tinctures away from light and heat.

***

Tips

1. Pick your herbs early in the morning just after the dew has dried.

2. You can leave the herbs in the alcohol for up to 6 months if you want to create very strong tinctures.

3. To make your tinctures doubly strong, you can pour the tincture after straining in step 5 above and store it for six more weeks.

4. Though the dose varies, a standard dose is 1 teaspoon diluted in water or tea and taken 1-3 times a day.

*****

Calendula Infused Oil

Equipment

Double boiler

Large glass bowl

Sieve and cheesecloth

Sterilized dark jars

***

Ingredients

16 fl oz. (500 ml) pure vegetable oil such as sweet almond oil or sunflower oil

8 oz. (250 grams) slightly crushed, dry calendula flowers or 16 oz. (500 grams) slightly bruised fresh calendula flowers

***

Instructions

1. Place the calendula and oil in the glass bowl ensuring that the oil covers the flowers. Simmer them in a double boiler for one hour at a temperature of around 120 degrees Fahrenheit (49 degrees Celsius). Do not let the oil and calendula boil. You can repeat this step several times after letting the oils cool to create more concentrated herb infused oils. You can make your oils even more concentrated by adding a fresh bunch of herbs with each re-simmering.

2. Strain the mixture through the sieve and cheesecloth into a clean, dark jar ensuring you squeeze out as much oil as you can from the herbs in the cheesecloth.

3. Label your jars with the manufacturing date, expiry date, herb and oils used.

4. Store your herb infused oils in a cool dark place or in the refrigerator and use them within 3 months.

*****

Calendula Salve

Equipment

Double boiler

Large glass bowl

Sterilized dark jars or tins

***

Ingredients

8 oz. (250 ml or 1 cup) herb infused vegetable oil (see previous recipe)

1 oz. (30 grams) beeswax

50 drops (2.5 ml or ½ teaspoon) essential oils like lavender essential oil

***

Instructions

1. Place the beeswax and herb infused oil in the glass bowl and melt them in a double boiler.

2. Once melted remove from the heat source and add the essential oils drop by drop until you get your preferred scent.

3. Pour the melted oils into the storage jars or tins and allow to cool completely.

4. Store the salves in a cool dark place.

***

Tip

If you want softer salves you can use less beeswax – for example ¾ oz of beeswax for 1 cup of vegetable oils.

*****

Calendula Lip Balm

Equipment

Double boiler

Large glass bowl

Lip balm tubes or small jars or tins

***

Ingredients

3 tablespoons herb infused vegetable oil (see recipe above)

1 tablespoon grated beeswax

1 tablespoon shea butter

***

Instructions

1. Place the beeswax, shea butter and herb infused oil in the glass bowl and melt them in a double boiler.

2. Once melted remove from the heat source and pour into lip balm tubes and allow to cool completely.

###

ABOUT THE AUTHOR

Marian Kim is an experienced alternative medicine practitioner.

*****

OTHER BOOKS BY THE AUTHOR

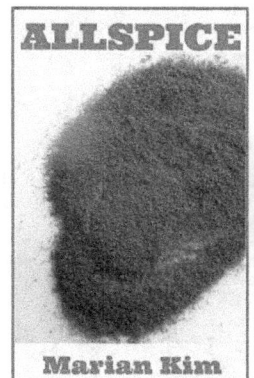

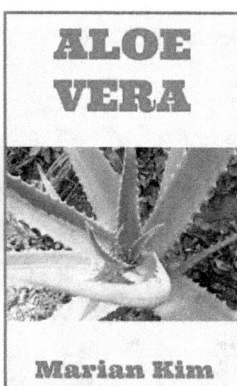

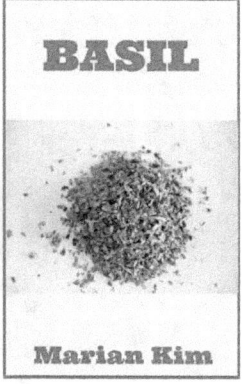

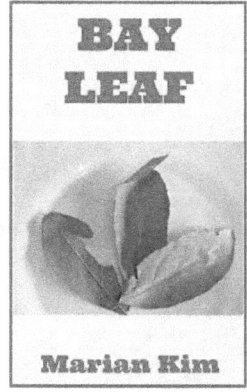

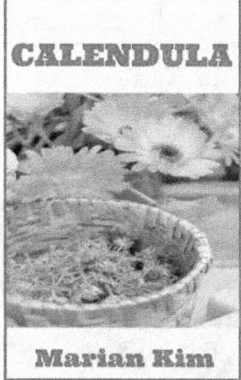

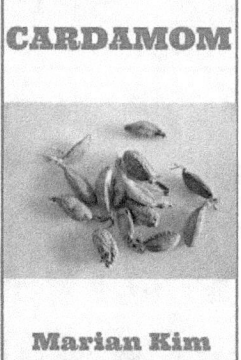

CAYENNE PEPPER

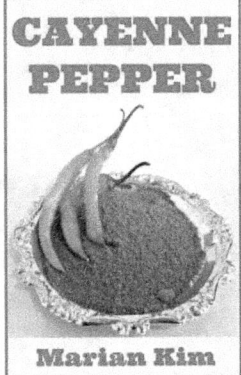

Marian Kim

CHAMOMILE

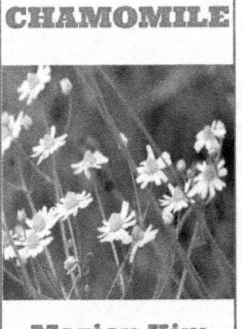

Marian Kim

CILANTRO & CORIANDER

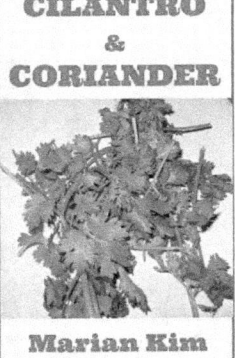

Marian Kim

CINNAMON

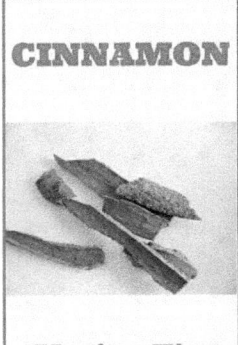

Marian Kim

CLOVES

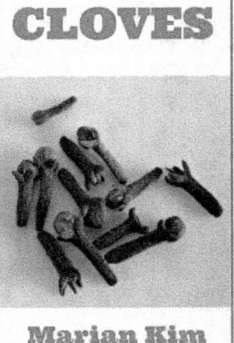

Marian Kim

CUMIN

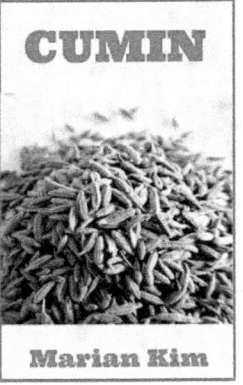

Marian Kim

DANDELION

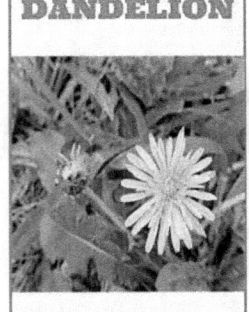

Marian Kim

DILL

Marian Kim

ECHINACEA

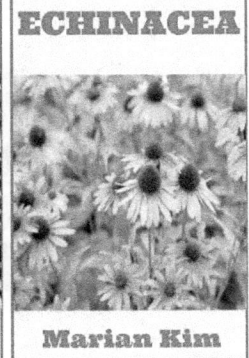

Marian Kim

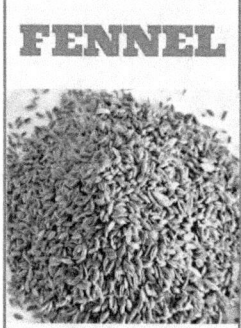

FENNEL

Marian Kim

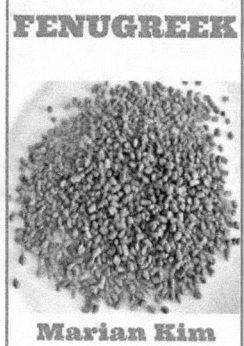

FENUGREEK

Marian Kim

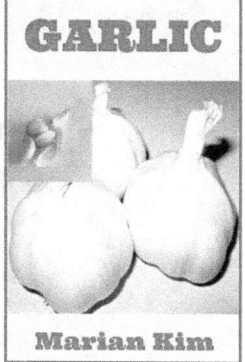

GARLIC

Marian Kim

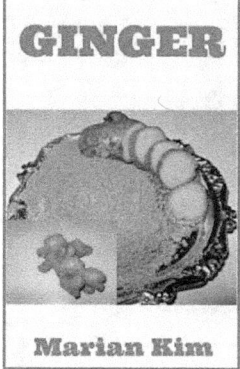

GINGER

Marian Kim

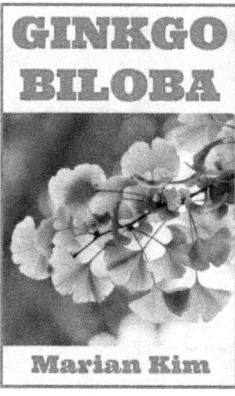

GINKGO BILOBA

Marian Kim

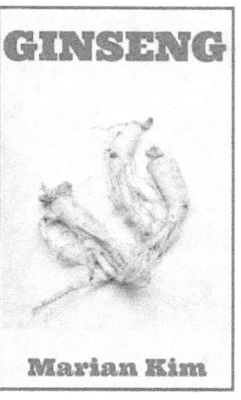

GINSENG

Marian Kim

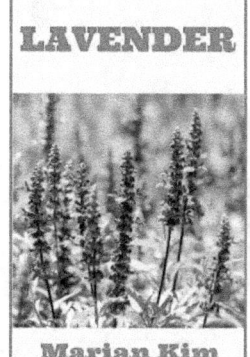

LAVENDER

Marian Kim

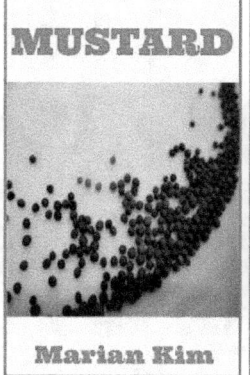

MUSTARD

Marian Kim

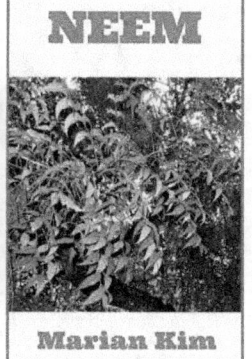

NEEM

Marian Kim

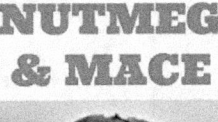

NUTMEG & MACE

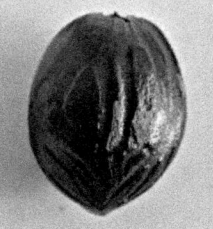

Marian Kim

OREGANO

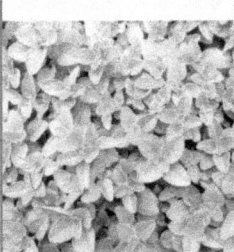

Marian Kim

PAPRIKA

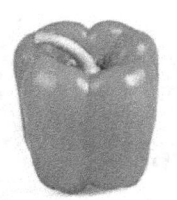

Marian Kim

PARSLEY

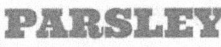

Marian Kim

BLACK & WHITE PEPPER

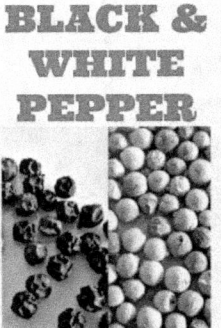

Marian Kim

PEPPERMINT

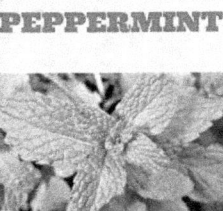

Marian Kim

ROSE HIPS

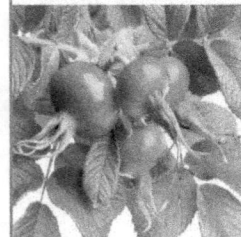

Marian Kim

ROSE PETALS

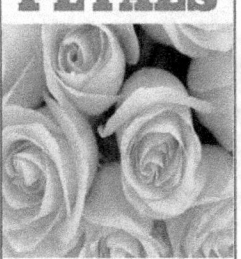

Marian Kim

ROSEMARY

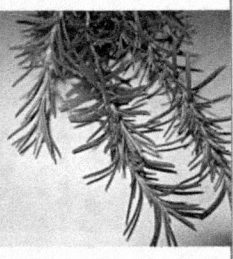

Marian Kim

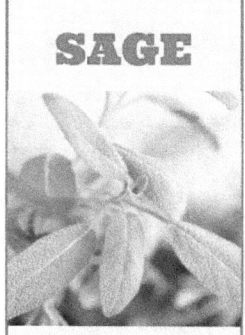

SAGE

Marian Kim

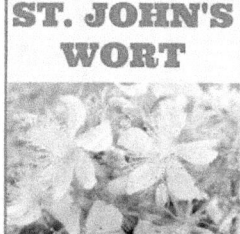

ST. JOHN'S WORT

Marian Kim

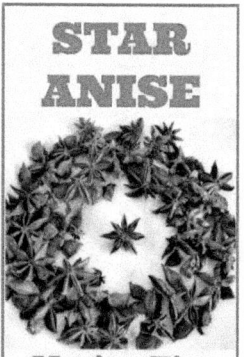

STAR ANISE

Marian Kim

STINGING NETTLE

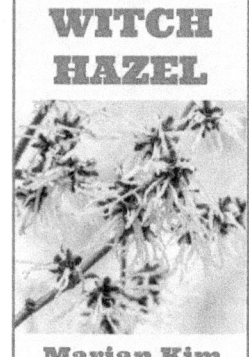

Marian Kim

THYME

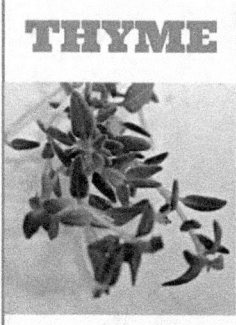

Marian Kim

TURMERIC

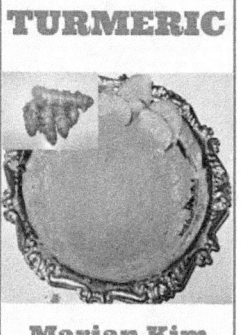

Marian Kim

WITCH HAZEL

Marian Kim

YARROW

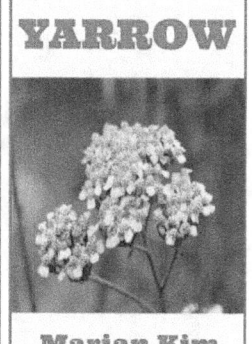

Marian Kim

*****

www.ingramcontent.com/pod-product-compliance
Lightning Source LLC
Chambersburg PA
CBHW071344310526
45790CB00018B/1358